Table of Contents

About the Cover

I cannot emphasize this enough, but once again, a huge thanks needs to go out to my friend, Christy Knutson. I don't know how she produces these great covers in the midst of her busy and productive life. Quite often, I give her the barest of ideas, and she produces the absolute highest work. I was thankful for her design on "Joy in Trials" and her work on both books in the "Which is Better?" series is phenomenal.

With this cover, she has done it again. In an eye exam, every patient sits in behind the phoropter and answers the "one or two" questions. So whether you are an Optometrist or some other business owner, this image fits the thought of the book perfectly.

Thanks again to Christy. Your help and concern is greatly appreciated. My readers thank you too, because once again, you saved them from having to look at my terrible cover creations.

If you want to find out more about her creations or perhaps hire her to help you out (which I would greatly encourage), you should check out http://www.moxiespeak.com/ or contact her at christy@moxiespeak.com.

Introduction

The small business landscape is being challenged. In fact, it might be in its most challenging age yet.

Salary demands are climbing, but quality staff are diminishing.

Governmental insurance demands make it more difficult to make a profit.

Specialized skills for your specific market niche are becoming harder to find, and when you do find them, employees want way too much money.

More and more folks are graduating from schools or colleges. There are less and less jobs. Oh, by the way, did I mention that many of these graduates have over $100,000 in school debt?

Business owners nearing retirement are finding it difficult to find anyone who can afford to buy their businesses.

It is not uncommon for a business to have six figures in outstanding credit card debt.

The bottom line is that Small Business Owners are just plain old tired.

And while no single book is going to address or solve all of these problems, this small book is intended to encourage you to enjoy your business once again.

To get you there, to help you enjoy walking in your office again, we are going to take an approach with which you might be familiar.

I'm sure you've been to an eye doctor before, but even if not, you've probably seen how doctors give eye exams. The place the phoropter in front of your eyes and ask, "Which is better: One or two?" That process is called a refraction. It determines a patient's eye prescription. Every now and then a patient may have 20/20, and if they do, they probably won't have it for long.
So, let's take that same approach to your business. Let's have an eye exam. Just like the Optometrist asks his or her patients, I'm going to ask you:

Which is better: One or Two?

What you'll find in the following chapters are three specific areas that if you apply the one or two model, you'll find an enjoyment in your practice, you'll find enjoyment with your staff, and you'll find enjoyment with your customers.

So, without any more waiting, here are your questions.

Which is Better: One or Two?

Whose Glory are You Seeking? Yours or the Business'?

Who Has to Be Right? You or the Best Idea?

What are You Zealous for? Profits or People?

Let's tackle these one by one, and along the way, we'll work through both good and bad examples. Then we'll give you an opportunity to work through the "one or two" yourself.

Enjoy.

Practice Progress, March 2013

Whose Glory are You Seeking?

Undoubtedly, you chose your specific industry because you were drawn to helping people with whatever specific skill or service you possess.

You love designing websites.
You love helping people.
You are a talented graphic artist.
You can repair a car like no one you know.
Fill in the blank.

And, without a doubt, somewhere along the line, you chose the industry you are in knowing that there was a good chance to make a decent wage, perhaps own a business, and you wanted the freedom to create the lifestyle that you chose for you and your family.

All of those things are perfectly fine.

The beauty of our country is the ability for folks to have a dream, seek it out, and see it come to fulfillment. So, wherever you are in that process, whether it be just graduating, working for someone else, or owning your own business, you are working towards the career that you want.

But there is a caution.

If your employees think that you are seeking your own glory as opposed to seeking what's best for the business, three things are going to happen.

Your business is going to suffer.
Your employee morale is going to be low
Your turnover is going to be high.

Seeking a successful career, building a successful business, and making money are fine, but they don't have to be synonymous with seeking your own glory. Let me explain.

Horrendous Example

I once knew a young man directly out of college. He had access to money and was able to start a business within just a few months of receiving his diploma.

He was handsome.
His wife was pretty.
He owned a burgeoning business.
And the whole world knew it.

Despite the fact that he was a talented, despite the fact that he knew how to work with his customers well, and despite the fact that he paid a good salary, his employees couldn't stand him. The reason his employees didn't support him was because in the day to day, he was seeking for himself. And since his staff felt he received enough glory as it was, they weren't going to add any more.

At first, the young man was content to see the staff resign. He rationalized it by saying they weren't the right people anyway, so over the next six months, nearly all of his staff left for other jobs. Slowly he created a new staff that he interviewed and that he hired.

All good, right? No, his business flat-lined, and he had could not keep a competent staff. He could still make money because he had a very stable business, but he wasn't able to grow it into what he hoped.

The main reason is that the impression he gave his staff was, "This is for me. My glory. You can be a part of it, but it is mine."

Here is the thing. Seeking your own glory is for rockers and movies stars. It is not how to build a healthy business. You can make money doing it (or not), but you won't build something with other people, and quite often, what you do build, you'll build alone.

Glorious Example

I once knew an incredible guy. He owned a small business. He was great at what he did, he was a smart businessman, he cared for his customers, and his staff loved him.

Why?

The reason his staff loved him was that no matter how much he paid attention to the bottom line, he paid attention to his staff. He created an environment where his employees cared about the day to day of the office because they loved coming to work, they enjoyed each other, and they liked their boss.

He didn't have any problems with staff familiarity. What I mean is that no matter how comfortable they felt around him, they still respected him and followed his leadership.

You might think that is impossible. You might think that there is no way staff can like you, trust you, and confide in you while simultaneously respecting you and following your leadership.

But just because that is hard to create, it does not mean that it is impossible to create. In fact, let me give you the key to that type of office, and I'll warn you that implementing this is not going to be easy.

If you seek the welfare of your staff, if you share in glory and praise, if you share the profits and the props, if you do those things before you take the glory for yourself, you will have an office environment that grows, is stable, and is productive.

Can you personality do that? It won't happen overnight, and you quite honestly might have a bad mix with your staff, but the biggest questions concern whether you, yourself, can seek to share the glory instead of seeking it for yourself.

To help you get there, let me give you some examples and some programs you might implement. Some of these you may have seen in the prior Practice Progress book, but some of them are unique to this effort.
Look at them, study them, and think about implementing them. If your

struggle with them has anything to do with a desire to keep things like profits from your staff, you have great soul-searching ahead.

But if you see these ideas and think, "Yeah, that makes sense. My staff will love these, and they will help us grow," you might have found the path towards sharing glory instead of owning it for yourself.

That might set your office on a path that could transform your workplace into something you and your employees really enjoy.

Ideas to Get You There

Understandably, not every idea here will work for every business.   However, there are enough provided to give you choices for what best fits your office. Remember, the picture here is to set a tone in your office that says,

"We share in the struggles so that we share in the glory."

Without systems to share the glory, the default impression becomes,

"You share in the struggle so that I can share the glory."

So with that in mind, check out these ideas.

Bonus Systems

Deposit Bonus - This is an all staff bonus that directly helps you put money in your pocket while motivating your staff. Here is how it works. Create a 12 month chart from the prior year that lists what your deposits were for each month.

Then project 5, 10, 15, and 20% growth.

Affix a value for each employee if they meet this goal.

Before I show you an example, let me address a few fears. You may not want your employees to know your deposits, but I will say they already do. They have a sense of how much money your office takes in, and it is probably an overly-skewed sense. Go ahead and tell them the truth. For most of them, it will be a reality check.

Secondly, don't worry about paying out these bonuses. You only have to pay them out when your office improves its deposits from last year and the payout for most offices is only a tiny % of the extra money you have put in the bank. Let me demonstrate for you.

Deposit Goals – 20xx

Last Year Dep	5% ($100)	10%	($125)
15% ($150)	20% ($175)		

Jan	66,327 76,276	69,643 79,592	72,960
Feb	71,754 82,517	75,342 86,105	78,929
Mar	80,858 92,987	84,901 97,030	88,944
April	87,763 101,042	92,151 105,316	96,539
May	77,089 88,652	80,943 92,507	84,798
June	80,223 92,256	84,234 96,268	88,256
July	71,673 82,424	75,257 86,008	78,840
Aug	75,674 87,025	79,458 90,809	83,241
Sep	76,026 87,430	79,827 91,231	83,629
Oct	81,950 94,143	86,048 98,340	90,145
Nov	62,457 71,826	65,580 74,948	68,703
Dec	67,525 77,654	70,901 81,030	74,278

Okay, let's take this in. In January of last year, you deposited $66,327 with a staff of 5 people. With a 5% increase of deposits to $69,643, you will give each one of those staff $100. Do the math.

You deposited $3,316 more in that month than you did in the same time period last year. You paid out $500 in bonuses. The net for you is $2,816.

Let's say that in that same month you have killer growth and increase your deposits by 20%. Do the math. You deposited $13,265 more in that month than you did in the same time period last year. You paid out $875 in bonuses. The net for you is $12,390.

This is a win/win for you. When your month is chugging along, and you know that if you and your staff work just a little bit harder or they need a little motivation to sell or market (whatever it is you do), this is how you get them to where they need to be.

This is also where you need to be able to project mid-month how you are doing. If your staff is aware of these numbers and they know how to project, they motivate themselves. But your input and your awareness of the numbers always help as well.

For example, if it is day 15 out of 20 in the month, and the staff see that they are falling a bit short of receiving their 5% bonus, then they know that with a little extra effort, they can hit their numbers. I mean, what else is going to motivate them?

If you have two business days left to go, or even just one, what is going to motivate your staff to work hard on a Friday? Nothing really. In fact, without something like this in place, you'll notice your
Fridays becoming more and more light. Your encouragement to them with a desire to pay them their bonus helps them work harder.

I have seen this exact scenario take place. One time, I was at a doctor's office on a Friday morning. I knew that there were several openings in the afternoon. Two patients called in a row asking about available exams, and the response they received was that there were openings next week. I thought, "What about today?"

Well, without some motivation to hit a number like a deposit, I'm afraid people are going to default to what is easiest. But if the staff is working towards getting $100, those two phone calls will be a blessing (and worth somewhere around $600). If you don't see this motivating your staff, you probably need new staff.

But here is the thing, when your staff realizes that you are saying to them, "When I make money, you make money," they will begin to change their impression of you. It won't be just your kingdom or just about your glory. Collaboratively, the staff will see that they get to share in the overall success of the office, and you celebrate that fact with them by giving them a bonus.

Weekly Bonus – I think every front desk, technician, web designer, and whatever in your office should have a bonus system, and they are outlined for you in the first Practice Progress book. But I want to include at least two more bonuses before we discuss other ways to share the glory. Each office needs a weekly bonus to keep them motivated.

Weekly bonuses work the same way as the monthly bonus, of course. You improve over last year, you share in the glory.

Let's say that you have set a goal for your staff to sell 30 widgets per week and you need to find a way to spiff your staff. Since no employee is successful all alone, I encourage an all office spiff.

Pick 4-5 affordable restaurants around you and make lunch the spiff. A great way to start a Monday is eating the lunch earned on Friday. And again, the cost is no big deal. Pizza, subs, etc are going to run you $50 or so for lunch. Your staff sold $X worth of widgets. In the long run, if your staff is consistently making sales, $50 worth of pizza is no big deal.

An added bonus is that sharing the spiff with the whole staff will improve inter-office relations. No matter how hard you have worked to protect salary anonymity, your staff assumes that somebody makes more money than they do. I've seen this turn really ugly before. The front desk person who gets to eat subs because the seller did their job well has one less thing to complain about.

Scheduling Bonus – If your office is a schedule based office, one of the most effective bonuses to motivate your front desk is how full they keep your schedule. For this to have its largest impact on your bottom line, you are going to have to monitor it well. Let me explain.

I recommend a spiff based on a % of your schedule being filled. For example, if you are an office with a healthy customer base, you may be scheduled out for a week or so at the time. That is a great problem to have, and you want to address that problem by seeing as many appointments in one day as you can. So, pick a % that is going to make your staff work hard and efficiently. For sake of demonstration, I'm going to choose 95% as the goal.

You can choose whatever you think will make your staff work hard but it also must be reachable.
To get to 95%, several things need to be in place. First and foremost, there has to be a schedule template (find those in

the original Practice Progress). Staff must be instructed as to where and when they place exams, office visits, follow ups, or whatever it is you schedule.

Never leave your schedule template to the whims of your front desk person or secretary. Though they may mean well, without motivation and accountability, your staff is always going to schedule as to what is convenient for them.

Without a template, you will almost never have a full schedule at the end of a day, and I guarantee you that you won't have busy schedules on Friday afternoons. Your job is to tell the front desk where and when to schedule; their job is to fill that schedule.

When they hit 95% (or whatever % you choose), you are working harder and they are enjoying a bonus. Spiffs for your front desk can be made up of a various items, but I like to go food for weekly and money for monthly. If 95% occupancy is your goal on a 3 appointments an hour schedule, then the entire office gets lunch if you have 3 appointments every hour all week 95% of the time. If you already have a lunch scheduled for Monday because of another department hitting their goal, great, then the staff gets lunch Monday and Tuesday.

A monthly spiff is easy to come up with; just remind yourself of the additional income you are enjoying because of the fuller schedule. But the takeaway for the staff is shared glory. Shared glory means a motivated staff and a healthy (mutually accountable) staff environment.

Complements

You might think, "Really, giving a complement is the best you can come up with?" But there is this reality. Many business owners do not complement their staff, and a result, the staff feel like they are working in a despotic kingdom.

This might be the hard part, but hopefully not. The complements have to be real, sincere, and based on something specific.

If your spouse asks you how something looks, and you say, "Good," that rarely gets it done. If you really like it, you would say, "That shirt complements your eyes," or "I can really tell you've been working out when you wear that." That gets it done. So, sharing glory with your staff is about specific complements.

If your customers work with you and your staff, then the handoff is the perfect time to give a complement. When you hand a customer off to an employee, tell the customer how well they are going to be cared for by that person. Tell the customer about a specific time your employee went above and beyond.

When you tell a customer that your secretary is going to schedule their next meeting, tell them (in front of that staff) that there is no one better at finding the perfect time for appointments than your scheduler.

You see, complements to your staff are effective, but sometimes, complements about your staff to the customer in front of the employee go even further.

If you can say these things honestly about your staff and with sincerity, you will be sharing glory with your employees. They will appreciate you more, work harder for you, and hang in there during the tough times.

Now for some questions to help you get there.

Questions to Help You Get There

Ask yourself the hard question, "Do you seek your glory before everyone else at your office?" Give yourself specific examples to support your conclusion or ask someone you trust.

How would your staff respond if you started spiffing them or giving them more complements? What can you do to be specific in both of these areas?

Make a point to ask customers specific questions about your staff so you can complement them. Ask how their check in process (or whatever interaction they have had) went or ask them if anyone on staff went above and beyond. The answers might teach you who to keep, who to praise, and who to encourage.

Who has to be Right?

The second "which is better" to consider is the question, "Who has to be right?" In your office, who is it? Is it you or is it the best idea? I imagine your first response is, "Well, the best idea, of course."

I wonder if your staff would say the same thing.

One way to determine the answer to that question is for you to do some soul-searching. Ask yourself these questions:

How often do I ask the staff for their opinion?

When was the last time I made a policy change that came directly from staff input?

When was the last time a staff person approached me with an idea that I actually put into place?

You might be asking these questions and think, "Uh oh." It might have been years (or never) since you made some office-wide change that came from a staff. And just because you can think of one, that doesn't necessarily mean your staff feels comfortable approaching you.

You can begin to see that this question is directly related to the first. If your employees think you seek your glory first, then they won't offer ideas even if you ask for them. If your staff feels like the glory is shared, then they will feel comfortable approaching you with innovation and change that will benefit the practice.

No matter how profitable or efficient an office is, once it stops innovating and seeking change and improvement, it begins to die. I have known quality employees who have left, even for less money, because they just felt like cogs in a machine.

Make them part of the process, and watch your office grow in innovation together. So, which is better? One or two? Your idea or the right idea?

This leadership principle will always be true. Your employees will treat your customers like you treat them.

If your employees think that you don't care about them, if they think you don't want their input, if they think that all you are trying to do is despotically run your office, then ultimately, that is how they will treat your customers.

They will be mad when customers don't have all their information.

They will abuse customers who owe money.

They won't be sympathetic to customers who have questions.

They will see the customers exactly like you see them: the thing that has to be dealt with in order to get a paycheck.

But if you create an environment where the best idea wins, then you will have a staff that is empowered and cared for. That staff will go above and beyond for your customers because you have gone above and beyond for them.

Let's look at some examples.

Horrendous Example

I once visited a business that was incredibly inefficient. Their secretary/admin staff didn't have clearly designated roles, and as a result, there was often a back-up of customers. Between customers walking in, filling out paperwork, shopping, checking out, and the host of other events that happened up front, a war was taking place.

It appeared that everyone who was working thought what they did was the most important and that every other task was someone else's responsibility. At times, factions of staff would gang up on others and treat them horribly as if there was an "in" crowd.

The wounded in this war were the customers. They were experiencing terrible service, they often waited forever to be helped, and their interaction with the employees could at best be described as curt.

The problem was not poorly trained or inexperienced staff. The problem was their understanding of roles and a clearly defined customer flow.

Now, the owner knew there was a problem. Customers complained and employees complained. As a result, the owner complained. The owner would gather the staff, voice his complaints, and even make threats to job security.

So, one day, an employee meekly approached the office and asked for a short sit-down. Understanding that the problem was a knot that needed to be untied, this employee had broken down the individual tasks (answering the phone, selling, cashier etc), and then assigned those tasks in terms for primary, secondary responsibility.

It was an incredibly well thought out answer to the solution. It didn't have to be THE solution, but it was well thought out.

Unfortunately, it wasn't received well. You see, this owner had a thing against assigned tasks. He felt that once you assigned tasks, no one helped out when others needed it. He felt that it bred a sense of, "That's not my job."

Now, the owner's viewpoint is understandable, and his concern about staff not helping each other out is valid in some circumstances. He has every right to create the staff structure he wants.

So what did he do? He told the employee that he was adamantly against narrowly defined job descriptions and responsibilities and that he was never going to allow employees to be in situations where they were tempted to not help someone else out. He did thank the employee but sent her on her way.

Less than two months later, that employee was gone and the problem remained.

What could he have done differently? Well, two things.

He could have changed his philosophy or at least given this alternative philosophy a shot. Or he could work with the best ideas of this talented staff person to develop a thought-out solution to the mess.

Instead, what he got was an unchanged mess and the headache of replacing a talented employee.

Essentially, he told the staff, the best idea is my idea.

Glorious Example

But there was another time, I saw an owner get it right. This owner had several offices, all of which shared a central office for admin. Each office was to send their numbers in digitally at mid-day and at the end of the day. Also, the owner had a runner that would both pick up and drop off any paperwork that needed to be submitted. At times, orders from the offices awaited approval from the central office.

Chaos reigned. Everyone felt their orders and reports were priority, and the admin office felt like no one appreciated the work that they did. There was a clearly defined system in place that the owner had designed, but it just wasn't working.

So, here is what the owner did. He closed early one Friday and brought everyone together. He provided lunch and gave everyone time to relax and enjoy it. As the meeting started, he spent significant time telling each staff how they were valued and praised them for specific instances where customers had related compliments.

Then, he readily admitted that the present system was not working. He owned that it was his design, and that though it might have seemed best at the time, it wasn't best now.

He then addressed specific breakdowns in the system, encouraged the staff to own their own mistakes and failures, and then he assured them that they would work together to design an inter-office system that was both efficient and staff-friendly. He then reminded them that no matter what that new system looked like, it should serve the customer's best interest. That would mean sacrifice and partnership.

He then told them to begin thinking of ways in which the system could be improved, he gave them a way in which they could contribute ideas either personally or anonymously, and then he told them to go home and enjoy their weekend.

All of sudden, the staff was at ease. They felt affirmed. They felt like their concerns had been heard, and they were given avenues for their suggestions. They did indeed go home and enjoy their weekend.

It took several weeks, but eventually, that owner had a brand new system that was efficient, practical, and collaborative. His employees felt like the owner owned his part in the problem, and they owned theirs.

Egos were set aside, and efficiency and partnership led the day. This boss made it clear. It didn't have to be his idea. It just had to be the best idea, and his staff followed in both attitude and implementation.

Now, not every problem can be solved with a staff meeting, a lunch, and a confession. However, something must take place for your staff to know that you are approachable with new ideas.

Let's work through the following ideas to see if they might help you figure out that approachability.

Ideas to Get You There

Just like before, let's remember that not every idea here will work for every office. However, there are enough provided to give you choices for what best fits your business. Remember, the picture here is to set a tone in your office that says,

The Best Idea Works

So with that in mind, check out these ideas.

Regularly Schedule Staff Meetings

Now, this idea is by no means revolutionary. In fact, you might have regularly schedule staff meetings already. But ask yourself these questions:

Does your staff enjoy these meetings or dread them?

Does your staff collaborate with you at these meetings?

How could you organize them so that they are both celebratory of success and analytical of weakness?

Part of what will make your staff meetings productive is objective feedback. Provide a way for both employees and customers to give praise and feedback anonymously. That way, the thanks and the thoughts can be worked through safely.

And if you do not have regularly scheduled staff meetings, consider them. If they aren't expected, then the ones you do have will fill your staff with a sense of dread. They'll think they are only called together to address problems.

And please provide food. The $50 you spend on pizza will be well worth it.

Reward Ingenuity

Let your staff know that you want them thinking and coming up with new ideas. Here are a couple ways to let them know.

Set up a process where new ideas can be submitted. You can have an inbox, an email address, or anything really. Just tell them in what form you want it, and then praise them for submitting good thought.

Give a flat fee for good ideas. Make it a formal application process. Anybody that submits an idea that makes your office more efficient or more profitable gets $100 cash. Pick whatever amount you want. The key is to make it enough for folks to care. Heck, offer an extra vacation day.

Regularly ask the staff, "Hey _____, got any good ideas for me today?" Remind them of what they have done. "You know _____, we were so much slower up front until you gave us that idea. Thanks so much."

Lead with Honesty

Be the first to admit when things are broken. And more importantly, be the first to admit that you own that breakdown. Yes, your staff plays a part, but you lead.

And be careful. Don't say, "Well, this is my fault because I let it happen, but I assure you this will never happen again." That sounds like you are blaming. Think along the line of, "Guys, I've let you down. You all work hard, and I should have either seen this problem coming or taken actions earlier. But I see now that this issue needs to be addressed, and I would like your help."

It goes so much smoother that way.

Now, after saying all that, here are some questions to help you process these things in your specific offices.

Questions to Help You Get There

What are areas of weakness in your office? How long have they been weak, and what are the causes of that weakness?

How can you own the weakness to your staff without it sounding like you are ultimately blaming them?

What is the simplest way to begin gathering in innovative ideas from your staff?

What would be reward your staff? Food? Money? Paid time off?

Where are areas where you gave the impression to the staff that you didn't care for their input? What are ways to address how that came across to your staff?

What is a neutral area, like marketing, that you could create a program where the staff could collaborate together to demonstrate that you value their thoughts and their input?

What are You Zealous for?

Let's be honest. You have to make a profit, and it surely isn't easy to do these days. If you aren't trying to make a profit, you most likely won't.

But it feels counter-intuitive to think, "If I give the best customer care in the city, we will ultimately make a profit." That thinking is hard because you know there are a million other areas to deal with:

Insurance
Staffing
Continuing Education
Taxes
Emails

And, I imagine you are doing your best to give the customer service possible.

But along the way, it is very easy to slip into a mentality that tries to see as many customers in a day as possible. There is nothing wrong with trying to maximize your schedule. But if you are just setting them up and then knocking them down, your customers will feel like cattle being run through the chute at the state fair.

Your challenge is to see as many as possible while still giving as much customer attention and care as possible.

Most of the difference comes down to your attitude.

And though I know that you want to give the best, highest, most proficient customer care in the most efficient way, it is still easy to slip into bad habits of rushing your folks out the door (or off the phone).

The few minutes that you take to invest in them and ask about them will make an incredibly difference in their perception of you. The moments you take to ask them how their office experience has gone will let them know that you care about how everyone is caring for them.
Again, I'm sure this is who you are and who you strive to be, but it is still something of which you have to be reminded of every now and then. Set out to be the best version of the boss/owner you dreamed of being in

school/training and don't settle for anything less.

Because if you don't daily remind yourself, both your customers and your employees are going to begin to think that all you care about is money. Again, you have to make a profit to stay in business and employ folks and care for folks. But the attitude that will create the most good will and the greatest longevity for your career is people over profits.

So, let's explore some bad and good examples.

Horrendous Example

I once knew a business owner who was rocking and rolling and making a good bit of money. Her employees liked her, and her customers loved her. She owned a business that was by appointment only. For the sake of anonymity, let's say it was a high-end salon. Either way, place yourself in her shoes. She was working on a schedule where she could see 3 customers in an hour, and she was seeing over 20 easily every day. The math was easy. With a no show here and there, she was seeing close to 400 every month.

As she and her staff conferred, they realized that with an adjustment of the work procedure and a slight shifting of responsibilities, they could get to 4 appointments an hour. Again, maximizing the schedule and making a healthy profit is a good thing.

But then something happened that no one expected. This incredibly gracious, conscientious business owner began to pay more attention to profits than to customers. Yes, her customer demand could easily fill 4 exams per hour. Yes, her staff could get them processed efficiently. And yes, the owner could see that many customers in an hour.

But she lost the sense of caring that her customers loved. Those 5 minutes that she lost meant a lot to her customers. They had less time to chat, and when she did find a customer that needed extra attention, they got less of her time there as well.

For a couple of months, the profits were booming.
The staff were digging the bonuses they were getting.
And the customers hated it.

Finally, a customer told her the truth. On a follow up appointment, this longtime customer just said, "You know, I don't know what it is, but the salon just feels different. Busier I guess."

This gave her pause.

Then, she discovered a long time customer was visiting a rival salon in town. So, she called her. The customer said the office just felt too busy for her, so she decided to find some place smaller and more intimate.

So the owner began randomly asking customers about their salon experience. Many answered the same way.

It was busy.
They felt rushed.
They missed the laid back feel.

After a few weeks of this, the owner just didn't know what to do.

The money was nice.
The profits were larger.
Her staff could handle the strain.
She enjoyed the quarterly owner distribution.

But in the end, her office was becoming something she never wanted. Her office had become the fast food restaurant of salons. And the dirty little secret was that she didn't know if she wanted to keep working this way.

Glorious Example

So, I bet you know where this is going? The glorious example comes from the owner who went to 4 appointments an hour. She made a bold choice. She went back to 3 appointments.

She didn't announce it to her patients, but she did to the staff. Here is what she did.

At her regularly scheduled staff meeting, she asked the staff how they thought the adjustment to 4 appointments an hour was going. While most of the staff thought it was going well, she sensed something that was going unsaid. She sensed they were tired, but no one actually said it.

Whether or not, she went ahead with her plan. She said, "Gang, you guys have been awesome. You have rocked and rolled, and we are seeing 4 appointments an hour as easily as we saw 3. I'm proud of you. Numbers and profits are up, and you guys just plain rock."

So far the staff was loving it.

Then she said, "But I'm afraid I have made a mistake. Though you guys are more than able to see 4 appointments in an hour, I'm afraid seeing that many is causing us to lose our identity. We just can't give customers the care we once gave them. In fact, I know that we have lost a few customers. Making money is nice, but I fear that if we keep this up, we are going to start losing more and more. This pace just isn't our office. So I've decided to go back to 3 appointments an hour."

At first her staff groaned. They enjoyed the bonuses they received for the office profitability, but once they made the adjustment, and once the office regain its own pace, they came around. In fact, a couple of staff told the owner that they thought it was the right decision, and at the next monthly staff meeting, everyone agreed.

Now, this story is not a parable about the dangers of seeing 4 appointments verses 3 an hour. That choice is for you to decide based upon your staff and your office philosophy.

The point of the story is that this owner realized that the move from 3 to 4 changed the nature of her office. No matter what she said, for her office, the changed emphasized profits over people.

The brave owner realized that making quick profits now would ultimately mean poorer customer care and perhaps fewer profits in the future. Her willingness to admit the mistake to her staff helped her regain some respect that she had lost.

And true story: she called that customer back. She explained that her office was seeing fewer customers per hour, and she came back.

People before profits.

You'll never regret it.

Ideas to Get You There

Understandably, not every idea here will work for every office. However, there are enough provided to give you choices for what best fits your office. Remember, the picture here is to set a tone in your office that says,

"Patients come before profits."

So with that in mind, check out these ideas.

Examine your schedule

Remember, 3 is not the magical number, and 4 is not the evil number. If you are a scheduled-based office, the right number for you should be the one that lets you optimize the schedule for customer care and profitability. That may mean adding an appointment or two throughout the day or it may mean cutting out a few.

Included in that is the question of whether you have the staff for the right schedule. Figure out the best schedule for your customer that your staff can handle. Train them towards greater efficiency and reward them for their improvement.

Staffing

Speaking of staffing, when you interview staff, how much do you quiz them about their customer interaction and experience? Also, you can tell so much about a staff person from their interaction with you and with their staff. Do this:

Bring your staff in and let them get to know each other. Ask the interviewee about specific times that they have dealt with an upset customer. Again, you'll learn a lot.

And when you give job reviews, how much of it has to do with customer interaction? Do you keep a record of when customers give praise or complain about a specific employee? Either way, staff need to be aware that they too are accountable for how well they care for customers.

Keeping Track of Your Customers

Many of you may have already gone paperless, so whatever your system it, this is a great way to keep up with your customers. It is nothing amazing or groundbreaking, but it works. You ready? Take notes. Here is what I mean.

On your customer's folder or in the file on the computer, keep track of their lives. I knew one owner who kept great notes on the outside of the file. It would read:

Loves dogs.
Just had another grandchild.
Misses her mother.
Used to live up North.

Whatever. The point was, the owner kept up with these details. So, right before he would meet with the customer, he would look over his notes. He would come in, greet them, and either during the appointment or at the end, he would ask follow up questions.

"So, how are your dogs? Wasn't one of them sick?"
"How are those grandbabies?"

"How are you and your family doing now that it has been a year since your mom died?"
"Have you taken any trips back North lately?"

And inevitably, the customers loved it. They just couldn't believe that the owner remembered all of these things. And the point was, he didn't, but he kept good records, and it helped create a bond with his customers.

Ideas for loving your customers are endless.

Emails on their birthdays.
Personal follow up calls after appointments.
Walking them to check out.

The point is, if you take extra care to care for your customers, your customers will insure that you make a profit.

Questions to Help You Get There

How can you begin gathering in honest feedback about your office? Could you approach some of your long time customers with a simple question or two that might inform you? Ask customers:

> Do you feel like we give you enough attention when you are here?

> Where are areas of the office that make you feel rushed or perhaps there is a bottleneck?

> Have you noticed any changes in the attitudes of the staff?

What is the maximum numbers of appointments your office can handle in an hour? Does that number lend itself to quality customer care? Why or why not?

Where are places in the day where you can redeem time, and where are places in the day where you can redeem time with customers?

Check yourself. Are you still giving customers the kind of time you gave them when you first began opened shop? Another way to say it is: Are you caring for customers in the same way you intended to when you were in school/training?

The hardest question of all: Are you brave enough to put the changes in place that will address the concerns you discovered in the previous questions?

Recap

So, there you have it. Your practice and your individual business philosophy have just walked through a comprehensive eye exam of sorts.

So, which is Better: One or Two?

Whose Glory are You Seeking? Yours or the Business'?

Who Has to Be Right? You or the Best Idea?

What are You Zealous for? Profits or People?

If you walked through the exam and discovered that you have 20/20, rock on. You are running your business the way that you always wanted to, you are creating an office environment that equips and partners with your staff, and you are giving quality of care the priority over blind profits.

But just like anyone with 20/20, I bet there are still a few issues to address. A 20/20 patient still needs to address issues of hydration, sunglasses, and contact lens. There are still areas you might want to tweak, so make your office and your personal business even better.

But more than likely, just like the majority of eye exams, your office probably doesn't have 20/20. It may not be cataract surgery time, but more than likely, there is a need for some corrective lens. Be brave. Address the issues with your staff, gather in input, and make the changes necessary. And just like you would advise your customers, don't wait. Make those corrections today.

Ultimately, seeking glory together as an office, seeking the best idea, and seek the care of your customers first will enable you to have an office that you enjoy walking into each day.

Be brave. Make change. Enjoy your practice.

One Final Note

Thank you so much for taking the time to read this book. It has been born out of a million mistakes, and I hope that it enables you to avoid the ones confessed to here.

As an old mentor use to say, "Mistakes are okay. Just make brand new one and avoid the old ones."

If there is ever any way in which I can help you or refer you to other resources, don't hesitate to contact us. You can always find more information at http://www.practiceprogress.com or at our Facebook page.

You can always email us at gordon@practiceprogress.com.

Also, please check out our releases:

Practice Progress – How to Maximize Eye Care Revenue

TeleTivoNetting – Accomplishing More by Doing Less

Praise for the Practice Progress Systems

Practice Progress

"This book should be gifted to every graduating O.D. today. Being an eye doctor is fun but being a businessperson is hard work. Gordon has the incredible ability of making the business of eye care easy and profitable." Jon Scott, OD

TeleTivoNetting

"If you're looking for a book (or rather pamphlet) that will help you process through your life and day in such a way as to become more productive and efficient with your time while not `over-doing' it or burning out then you'll find this book beneficial and challenging for you. It's full of questions that help you evaluate the things you do. Gordon cuts through much of the fluff that you often find in books like this and get's to what you really desire. I found myself thinking through the things I do with a critical eye seeing how I could be more effective, efficient, and restful person." Jeremy G

About the Author

Gordon Duncan is an award-winning educator, salesman, teacher, manager, and writer. He has taught in the public school system, lobbied for school's accreditation, managed eye clinics, led sales' teams, and also publishes books on theology, church, and culture.

In addition, he writes regularly on running and spiritual issues through http://www.examiner.com/evangelical-in-raleigh/gordon-duncan,and http://www.examiner.com/running-in-raleigh/gordon-duncan.

You can find out more about his philosophies for the eye industry at www.practiceprogress.com and his thoughts on church and culture at www.jgordonduncan.com.

He has been happily married to Amy for over 15 years and is the proud father of 3 wonderful girls.

He is a graduate of East Carolina University and Reformed Theological Seminary.

Which is Better: One or Two?

www.ingramcontent.com/pod-product-compliance
Lightning Source LLC
Chambersburg PA
CBHW051245170526
45165CB00004B/1577